HANDBOOK
OF A
PARENT!

Dr. Humeraa Qamar
MD, MPH, FAAP

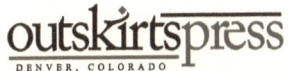

outskirtspress

DENVER, COLORADO

Outskirts Press, Inc.
http://www.outskirtspress.com

ISBN: 978-1-4787-6660-5

Outskirts Press and the "OP" logo are trademarks belonging to Outskirts Press, Inc.

PRINTED IN THE UNITED STATES OF AMERICA

Table of Contents

Introduction

Congratulations would-be parents and parents!

You have found the perfect handbook to help navigate parenthood. As a practicing pediatrician, a mom and hoping to be a grandma soon, I want to help you to the best of my ability in that most momentous of a task: raising a happy, healthy child. Contrary to what most people believe and propagate, parenthood is not an exact science. It is a lot of hits and misses and intuitive actions. Simultaneously, it's fun and extremely fulfilling. However, it is true that having a reliable simple guide will make your job easier. This is where my book will come in handy as I pen a treatise that I hope you will turn to over and over and over again. I have made an effort to keep it concise and easily readable.

For ease of understanding I have divided my book into chapters that will coincide with how visits to my office are set up. From prenatal to first, second, third… visits, all the way to age twenty-six. This volume will be dealing with wellness visits. The second volume of the book will deal with some common childhood illnesses and developmental issues that I see in my practice. The most important thing I tell my parents is that the milestones we discuss during various visits are generalizations and each child is unique in how and when she develops. It is good for parents to educate themselves about these things and always discuss with their pediatricians any perceived deviations. Parents are pediatricians' best allies in caring for their children. I tell my parents that they are my eyes and ears, and I work with them as a team to ensure optimum health and development for my little patients.

1

Prenatal visit.

Congratulations! You have just found out that you and your partner are expecting! (I am going to use the word partner instead of husband and wife for the most part as it is most reflective of the current family milieu). It is a scary yet exciting moment. After the initial dust settles, your obstetrician and friends and family will tell you to find a doctor for the baby, that gentle soul who will be your partner in raising your child: THE PEDIATRICIAN. I usually recommend that you look around, ask friends for recommendations whose kids already go to pediatricians' offices, ask your obstetrician and make a list of possible doctors. It is also a good idea to check your insurance website for pediatricians covered by your insurance. Once you have a few names picked out, call the offices and see if they offer prenatal visits. Almost all pediatricians offer complementary prenatal visits. You should be definitely going in for this prenatal visit, not only to meet the doctor but also to meet the staff and check out the cute, clean offices. Make a list of questions before you go in that can be asked during a 10-15 minute visit (sorry, guys, no prenatal visit is an hour long). Some of the questions that you might want to ask are: Are same-day sick visits available? Procedure for circumcision (if it is a boy), how quickly will you get call backs from the nurses, what is the average wait time in the office? Are they offering all the childhood vaccines currently recommended by the American Academy of Pediatricians? While you are there you can mingle with the patients in the waiting room and ask how satisfied they are with the office, doctors and staff. Note the general atmosphere and cleanliness of the office. Once the prenatal visits are done you and your partner can choose the doctor that appealed to you most and give that name to your Ob's office. That way when you deliver at the hospital, the nurses in the nursery will know who to call to notify of the baby's arrival.

Here is what I discuss and recommend to my expectant parents during the prenatal visit:

First and foremost is the important recommendation of breast feeding the baby. Contrary to what they show in videos and movies, breast feeding is hard work for both the baby and the mom. To be successful, it requires a lot of patience and perseverance (especially with your first baby). Moms and their partners need a lot of encouragement and ongoing support in the first few weeks. I usually recommend that parents attend prenatal classes offered by the local hospitals. If you are having a boy then it is important to discuss with the pediatrician circumcising the baby. I usually recommend circumcision as circumcised baby boys have less incidence of urinary tract infections and other infections in childhood and adulthood and are definitely easier to clean. Other stuff that I want parents to get, in addition to whatever else they deem appropriate, is a cool mist humidifier, rectal thermometer, a good breast pump and baby nasal saline to be used as needed on the baby under the pediatrician's guidance.

2

Stork brings the baby.

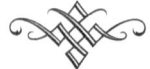

While it is true that some families choose unconventional deliveries at home by nurse midwives, more than 95 percent of babies get delivered at hospitals by nurse midwives or the obstetricians. Once the baby is born in the delivery room, make sure the nurses know that you (the mom) want to keep the baby with you for at least an hour (unless, of course, the baby needs immediate medical attention in which case the baby will be taken to the newborn nursery right away). The first hour after delivery is when the newborn is most awake and active. This has been labeled as the golden hour by nurses, pediatricians and lactation specialists, as this time is the most conducive to maternal/baby bonding and breast feeding. So after the nurses or the doctor quickly dry and check the baby out, they will hand over the baby to the mom. Skin to skin contact is started and the mom, with the nurses' help should put the baby to the breast. Even if the baby latches on for a few minutes on each breast, it is sufficient to initiate the increased production of Prolactin (the milk hormone) which ensures the smooth and ongoing production of milk. In the event that the baby is born via a c section, the skin to skin contact and the initial latching on will get delayed. But, no matter, it can still be achieved afterwards, as soon as the obstetrician allows it. After this initial breast feeding session, the baby and the mom get moved to another room in the hospital where the mom will stay until discharge.

Most hospitals in USA have implemented the concept of Couplet Care in which the same nurse takes care of the baby and the mom, and the baby stays with Mom in her room. Very rarely does the baby leave the mom's room to go to the nursery. Of course, if the baby requires more intensive medical care, he or she will be taken to the nursery. Your doctor will let you know if that happens. For a normal vaginal delivery, the mom and the baby will stay in the hospital for forty-eight hours. For c section deliveries, the length of stay is usually three days. During that time the baby's doctor will visit and examine the baby every day and discuss care and issues with the parents. Again, any change in the baby's care may lengthen the stay. During the baby's stay the baby gets eye ointment to prevent any possible eye infection, intramuscular Vitamin K injection to prevent bleeding disorder, Hepatitis B vaccine, hearing screen and a test called the PKU. This PKU test checks for several congenital diseases which if picked up on time are totally curable. This test checks for protein digestion, red blood cell disorders like sickle cell disease, thyroid disorders, etc. to name a few. If everything is normal in this test you will not hear anything from the state or the pediatrician. If something shows up abnormal on this test you will receive a letter from the state health department, your pediatrician will notify you, and appropriate follow up will be scheduled. Each state has a slightly different panel and is done free of cost on all newborns. If the parents are doing a home delivery I recommend that the nurse midwife performs all of the above on the baby, including the PKU test. Similarly, if the baby fails the hearing screen at the hospital, a follow up appointment will be given to repeat the test. If you have a baby boy and want the baby circumcised this is the best time to ask the pediatrician to do it.

A significant number of babies develop yellow discoloration of the eyes and the skin or jaundice about a day after birth. This happens because when the baby is inside the mom the baby breathes through the mom's placenta and hence requires a large amount of red blood cells to extract the oxygen from the mom's placenta to carry it to the baby. Once the baby comes out and starts breathing on his or her own, the extra red blood cells get broken down and the one of the byproducts is the yellow pigment, bilirubin. Until the baby's liver catches up, bilirubin spills over into blood and causes jaundice. This physiologic jaundice peaks around the third day of life, never gets very high and then starts clearing up gradually. Usually the jaundice starts spreading from head down to the feet and starts clearing from feet upwards. Breast-fed babies can stay jaundiced up to six weeks after birth. Any cause of jaundice other than the normal jaundice will be dealt with by the pediatrician separately. If everything goes well the baby should be discharged according to the above schedule. Upon discharge make sure the nurses write down for you the discharge weight of the baby, which will be less than the birth weight as all babies normally lose weight for a few days after birth. Most pediatricians want to see the baby within three to five days after discharge from the hospital. If you have a home birth the baby will need to be seen within twenty-four hours after birth.

3

Baby's first visit to the pediatrician.

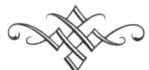

As mentioned above, the baby needs to be seen within 1- 4 days after birth. The main purpose of this visit is to weigh and examine the baby and check on mom to see how she is doing. The pediatrician does a thorough physical exam on the baby in front of the parents and goes over the baby's care and feeding at length with them. It is important to also check on the mom's health and well-being; a happy, healthy mom will lead to a happy, healthy baby. I usually ask about the social/physical support system available to the mom, including that of the partner and both sets of grandparents to ensure a smooth transition. Some moms can suffer from postpartum depression after the baby's birth, which is easily treatable if identified correctly. The baby's doctor and Mom's doctor should work together as a team for this.

The baby's weight in the office is compared with the baby's discharge weight from the hospital to ensure that the baby is gaining adequate weight. As a rule of thumb half an ounce to one ounce per day for breast and one ounce per day for bottle babies is considered adequate weight gain. It is important to encourage mom and tell her that it is not uncommon for the baby to continue to lose weight for the first week, especially breast babies. For exclusively breast-fed babies, it is recommended to give the baby 400 International Units of Vitamin D drops per day, as sometimes mom's breast milk may not have adequate amounts of Vitamin D. The mom is encouraged to eat a healthy balanced diet and consume a lot of water to keep herself hydrated. I also recommend that the mom should avoid all dairy products and green leafy vegetables in her diet for the first couple of weeks. It is also advisable for the mom to avoid caffeine, alcohol and all medicines while breastfeeding, unless approved by the pediatrician. This is the visit when a baby's circumcision is healing and the umbilical cord is still oozing and gel-like, so it is recommended to not bathe the baby in water but to sponge clean with a clean soft, cotton cloth. After the above goals have been achieved, the baby will be brought back in two to seven days again to the office to ensure ongoing, adequate weight gain. A common question my parents ask me is how they can determine if they are feeding the baby the right volume, that is, not overfeeding or underfeeding the baby. A simple rule of thumb I tell my parents is that they need to remember that the size of a newborn's stomach on the first day of life is the size of a cherry (1-2 teaspoon), on day number three of life it is the size of a walnut(one ounce) , day number seven of life it is the size of an apricot (1.5 to 2 ounces) and by the time the baby is one month old it is the size of an egg (2.5 to 5 ounces). Beyond age one month it enlarges very slowly. Any amount greater than above given to the baby will make the baby throw up.

4

Here we come again! Second week visit.

The purpose of this visit is the same as the first one. Baby's weight gain and mom's health is assessed and a detailed question-answer session is conducted. The family is encouraged to not take the baby out in public, especially crowded areas like the grocery stores. The temperature at home should be maintained at around 74 degrees Fahrenheit and baby should be comfortably clothed in soft pre-washed cotton outfits. There should absolutely not be any smoking or pets around the baby. The baby should be sleeping in a crib or bassinet next to the mom's bed to ensure ease of breast feeding at night. Because of the risk of Sudden Infant death Syndrome (SIDS) the baby should always be put to sleep on his or her back (never on his/her tummy). Usually at this visit the cord has fallen off and the stump has dried up and for circumcised baby boys the circumcision has healed and the green signal can be given to the parents to bathe the baby in a safe bathtub on an even surface in a well lit room. The baby should never be left alone in the bathtub or any surface.

5

Cutie pie turns one month!

If all is going well with the baby's weight gain and the parents feel comfortable, the next visit will be when the baby turns four weeks old. In addition to checking the baby's weight, feeding techniques, volume, duration, etc. baby safety are discussed at length. Other things that can come up during this visit are clear discharge from the baby's eyes, which occurs because of obstruction of tear ducts. This is not an infection and responds well to massaging the tear ducts and clean warm compresses. If the eye gets red or the discharge becomes thick and pussy looking, the pediatrician needs to be consulted as it may be an eye infection. It is important to involve the spouses, grandparents and siblings in all visits, as they play an important role in the well-being of the baby and mom. I recommend not giving any medicines, including fever reducers like Tylenol or Ibuprofen to the baby, unless recommended by the pediatrician. Also a lot of babies may sound nasally congested for the first few weeks of life, as mom's hormones can cause some nasal swelling in the baby. The best remedy for this is to run a cool mist humidifier in the baby's room, especially at night, or use baby saline drops in the baby's nose in the form of 1-2 drops every 6-8 hours as needed. If the baby has difficulty breathing or runs a fever, call the pediatrician. The best way to check the baby's temperature is via a rectal thermometer. Any temperature greater than 100. 4 Fahrenheit is a fever for the baby and needs immediate medical attention.

Another thing that may come up in this visit is questions about bouts of crying that the baby experiences, usually in the evenings, that may last 2-3 hours and don't seem to be associated with anything in particular. This is called Colic, AKA parent worrier. Colic is not reflective of any disease for the baby. It is a phase the baby goes through, almost a mild overstimulation which the baby deals with by crying. It is definitely not indigestion. If your baby is doing this, gentle rocking may help. Discuss with the pediatrician during the next visit. Babies spitting up milk is a very common phenomenon and does not signify disease. All babies spit up, some more than others. This is because the baby's stomach is small and the valve between the food tube and stomach is leaky. The remedy for this is frequent burping and keeping the baby upright for half an hour after the baby is done eating. If the vomiting is frequent then I will sometimes try to change the formula or eliminate dairy from Mom's diet and give baby an antacid to help. As long as the baby gains good weight, we don't do any other intervention; the baby will outgrow reflux by the time the baby is more mobile and is sitting up more (usually between nine to twelve months old). If the vomiting becomes projectile or the baby loses weight, the pediatrician needs to examine the baby to rule out any obstruction in the gastrointestinal tract.

6

Vaccines start to keep the baby healthy!

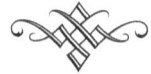

The next well checkup for the baby is the two-month-old well visit. This is the visit when the baby will start her/his first set of vaccines at the pediatrician's office. (The first vaccine that the baby received was the first hepatitis vaccine at the time of birth in the hospital). Vaccines are an extremely important part of your child's health and well-being and are 100% recommended by me and all health professionals. No study has ever shown that vaccines cause autism or any other neurological disorders. (Please refer to the attached vaccine schedule recommended by The American Academy Of Pediatrics for the list of childhood vaccines).

The baby's weight, length and head circumference is measured by the nurse and written for the parents in the baby's growth book. Babies will usually gain about 1-2 pounds weight, about an inch in length and half an inch in head circumference per month for the first six months of life. The baby should be breast feeding 15 minutes on each breast every 2-3 hours or consuming 2-4 ounces of expressed breast milk or formula via bottle every 2-3 hours. The baby should have about 6-8 wet diapers per day and poop after every feeding at breast or 1-2 times per day for formula babies. The stools for the formula babies will be brownish firm by this age and breast stools will still be yellow seedy, sometimes watery and explosive. Sometimes it seems like the baby is straining to poop and may turn red in face but the stool that comes out is soft. This is not constipation. It is hard for the baby to have a bowel movement when lying down. The baby must learn to squeeze his/her abdominal muscles and relax the anus in order for the stool to come out and this upsets the baby. Don't worry, usually by the time the baby is 3-4 months old the stooling becomes less stressful and easier for the baby. If the stool gets hard or contains blood, definitely call the pediatrician's office. Some of the other things I discuss with the parents during this visit are that most babies are making good eye contact and responding to human faces by smiling. The babies can start getting tummy time during the day for about ten minutes, or until the baby gets tired. The baby will still continue to sleep on her/his back, of course. One dose of baby Tylenol is given to the baby either before or after the vaccines. The baby may run a mild fever (99 or 100 degrees Fahrenheit from the vaccines). Fever is a good body response after the vaccines and we don't want to suppress it too much.

7

Look who is four months!

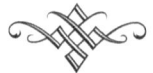

Things have settled down into a nice routine for the baby and the family by this point. This is the start of a very interactive phase for the baby. The baby smiles, coos, makes good eye contact, brings hands to the midline and sometimes rolls over at this age. After the usual growth measurements I inquire about the above milestones. For formula babies I recommend starting spoon feedings at this age. This is a slow process in which the baby will be spoon fed with single foods like a little rice or oatmeal cereal or fruits or vegetables. Only a couple of teaspoons per day for 2-3 days to make sure that the baby is tolerating the spoon feeding well. Parents can buy Stage 1 baby food (preferably organic) from the market or make it at home by boiling single foods and then straining and pureeing into soft consistency. I recommend no more than two ounces of baby food at each feeding. Once you have tried all single fruits and vegetables (no pineapple or strawberries, please) it is time to move the baby to breakfast, lunch and dinner spoon feedings. If you spoon feed two ounces baby food each time, it should be followed by four ounces of formula or breast milk after that. So the baby will be consuming six ounces of baby food per day plus about 26 ounces of formula per 24 hours. Total feeding (baby food and formula or breast milk combined) will then be 32 -34 ounces per day. For totally breast-fed babies, it is considered acceptable to wait until the baby is six months old to start this process. The baby starts to drool a lot around three months of age but the first teeth won't appear till the baby is between 6-7 months of age. The reason the babies start drooling at three months of age is because the salivary glands start developing, the teeth within the gum start moving up to the gum line in preparation for eruption and, most importantly, the saliva has digestive enzymes that help the baby digest the stage 1 foods. Most babies will double their birth weight by the time they turn four months old.

8

Yes, I am six months!

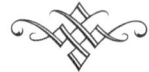

If everything goes well, the next well checkup for the baby is when she/he turns six months old. By this age the baby is rolling over both ways, sitting up with support, reaching for things, cooing loudly and sleeping about 6-8 hours at night. The baby makes good eye contact and laughs and is also babbling a lot. Some babies will be scooting backwards or rocking on their fours. Usually this is the age for breast fed babies to start on stage 1 baby food and for formula fed babies to move to Stage 2 foods. Stage 2 foods are more in volume (usually 4 ounces) and have more mix and match variety. Also now we can start the baby on proteins like chicken or turkey. No seafood yet. The baby will continue on the three meals a day regimen. For breakfast 2-3 tablespoons of cereal mixed with stage 1 fruits to make a total volume of four ounces around 7:00-8:00 a.m., a jar of stage 2 for lunch around 11:00 a.m. and a jar of stage 2 for supper around 5:00 p.m. Each meal of four ounces followed by two ounces of formula or breast feeding to give a volume of 32 ounces per day for the baby. This will be comprised of twelve ounces of spoon feeding and 20 ounces of formula or about five breast feedings. This provides adequate nutrition for growth and development for the baby. We can also start introducing the stage 1 sippy cup to the baby with some water in it. About 2-4 ounces of water per day is adequate. The baby will cut her first tooth between 6-7 months of age. In some babies the teething will get delayed up to nine months. Teething will make the baby irritable and the baby may run a low fever like 99 or 100 degrees Fahrenheit. Any fevers higher than 101 are not due to teething. The baby gets a headache and jaw ache which makes the baby pull at her ears. These symptoms look like those of an ear infection and you should take the baby to the pediatrician to differentiate. As soon as the first tooth erupts I recommend cleaning with a soft clean cloth. The earliest you can put sunscreen on babies is usually age six months. Even then, if you take the baby outside to someplace like the beach, the baby should wear a hat and long pants and sleeves and direct sun exposure should be restricted to no more than fifteen minutes.

9

Look Mom, I am a big baby!

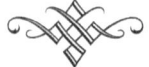

Before you know it the baby's 9-month-old well visit rolls around. The baby at this age will be sitting without support, crawling well, pulling up to standing position and taking a few steps while holding onto things (cruising). Some babies are even walking independently at this age. Independent walking is rare, so don't get upset if your baby is not walking yet. The baby starts saying 'dada' (most of the time this is non-specific and does not mean dad). Most babies have also developed pincer grasp in which they can hold small objects between their finger and thumb and try to put it in their little mouths. This is the age when we can move the baby to stage 3 foods and introduce soft, cut up table foods which babies can feed themselves. In addition to three meals a day, babies should be offered 2-3 healthy soft snacks a day which they can finger feed themselves. I recommend introducing hyper allergenic foods like cooked eggs, peanut butter and seafood at this age. Studies have shown that introduction of these foods before the baby turns a year old actually helps prevent food allergies in kids. Self-feeding and spoon feeding should be carried out in the baby's high chair. Self-feeding should always be done under an adult's supervision. The baby should be drinking about 16-18 ounces of formula per day or breast feeding about 3-4 times a day. The baby can also be given about ten ounces of water per day via a stage 2 sippy cup. No juices yet. The baby should not be given any night feeds and should be encouraged to sleep through the night. It is important for the baby's safety to child proof the whole house. Remember the rule: What you think your baby cannot do, he will do! The American Academy of Pediatrics no longer recommends giving children's Syrup of Ipecac to the baby to induce vomiting in case of accidental ingestion. Please put the phone number for the Poison Control Center at 2-3 prominent places around the house so you can call them if you find that the baby may have ingested something poisonous. Remember prevention, prevention, prevention!

10

First birthday cake!

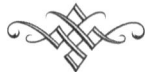

This is a big, emotional milestone for the whole family. As babies venture into their second year of life a lot of things are changing. They are not growing as fast as they did in the first year of life, so the appetite goes down and more independent eating habits kick in. This is a positive change and should be encouraged by the parents. This is the age to transition babies to all table foods and whole milk in a cup. This is the age to wean from pacifiers also. Prolonged bottle and pacifier usage, beyond the first year of life, has been associated with a lot of negatives. The baby can develop what is called milk bottle caries or rotten teeth. Prolonged sucking on bottles or pacifiers increases mal occlusion of the teeth causing negative changes in the shape of the roof of the mouth, which impairs proper growth of the mouth. It also increases the incidence of middle ear infections.

The baby is babbling a lot more and saying 2-4 words. Most babies start independent walking around this age (the average age for independent walking is thirteen months).

The baby should be offered ten ounces of water per day with a sippy cup. The baby should be transitioned to whole, vitamin D, preferably organic, milk in a cup. About 12-16 ounces of milk per day is enough. Remember too much milk can lead to anemia, protein deficiency and sometimes constipation. I don't recommend starting juice for babies until they are two years old. The baby should be offered three meals a day plus healthy cut up, soft snacks throughout the day. The baby has become very picky and should not be force fed. This is the age when we start the baby on multivitamins with iron. Until the baby gets the front molars it is best to use liquid multi vitamins. It is best to mix the dose in a couple of teaspoons of applesauce daily and feed to the baby. Don't mix the vitamins with milk, as calcium impairs the absorption of Iron. Once the baby gets the front molars, we can switch to chewable multi-vitamins with Iron. I don't recommend the gummy vitamins as they can stick in the baby's teeth or throat and can pose a choking hazard. Plus these vitamins don't have Iron in them which all children, especially toddlers, require to maintain healthy hemoglobin. The baby has about four teeth by this age. Fluoride is a vitamin which makes the enamel of the teeth stronger. If you don't have fluoride in the water that the baby drinks, talk to your pediatrician about supplementing Fluoride.

11

15-month visit.

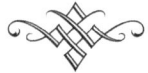

The next time we will see the baby for a well visit is when the baby turns fifteen months old. Ninety percent of the babies are walking by this age. The baby has improved her pincer grasp and can eat with a fork and spoon. The baby's picky eating pattern continues and baby should be offered three meals and small healthy snacks throughout the day. The baby should be drinking 12-15 ounces of organic, whole vitamin D milk and 10-12 ounces of water per day. The baby's vocabulary expands to about ten words. Ninety five percent babies are sleeping 10-12 hours at night without waking up. If the baby is waking up crying inconsolably at night with his eyes closed, the baby is having night terrors. These are normal for this age and all that is required is to check on the baby to ensure the baby's safety and leave the baby alone. It is not necessary to wake the baby up. The baby can also start having nightmares at this age. With nightmares the baby actually wakes up and cries consolably. Babies also develop separation anxiety at this age in which they start understanding that they are separate from mom and people exist when they are not present, something called object permanence. This makes them cry when they don't see Mom. This is a normal developmental stage and soon passes. Separation anxiety is different than stranger anxiety which typically starts around four months of age and peaks around fifteen months and dissipates around two years. Stranger anxiety manifests by the baby looking differently at strangers and crying and hiding behind Mom in the presence of a stranger. Gentle reassurance and gradual exposure makes both anxieties manageable.

12

18-month visit!

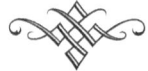

It is really gratifying for me as a pediatrician to see my 18-month-old toddler patient walk in independently into my office and not cry. Developmentally the baby is smiling, walking independently, stacking four blocks, and pointing to pictures. The typical vocabulary consists of ten words and baby will use single words to indicate needs. Most babies at this age will hold a crayon and imitate scribbling. Babies this age will smile at me and even give me high fives with Mom's help. Eating and drinking pattern stays the same as the 15-month-old visit. The baby can now eat skillfully with a fork and spoon. Some babies have become conscious of peeing and pooping sensations and will point to the diaper after soiling it. The baby sleeps about 10-12 hours at night and takes a 2-hour nap in the afternoon.

13

Independence, thy name is second birthday!

The two-year-old toddler continues to develop exponentially. This is the age of the "terrible twos" when the baby has major temper tantrums. These tantrums arise as baby understands a lot more than what he can express and hence gets frustrated. The important thing to understand is that this is a normal development stage and does not need to be suppressed or punished. The best approach is to ignore the temper tantrums. The less attention you pay the sooner the baby snaps out of it.

The baby's speech has taken off to about thirty words. The baby can put two single words together, like me go, me want etc. The baby is able to follow two step commands like, "Go to the next room and fetch a diaper." The baby can stack more blocks and go up and down steps. The baby's fine motor skills continue to evolve. He is able to use eating utensils very well for feeding.

Baby should be eating three meals a day and several healthy snacks throughout the day. The baby should drink two cups of 2 % organic, vitamin D milk per day and about ten ounces of pure water per day. We can start to offer about 4-6 ounces of calcium fortified orange juice to the baby at this age. The baby can still only play by herself and is not able to share her toys. A lot of parents ask me about the ideal age to put the baby in a day care. I usually recommend waiting, if they can, until the baby turns two years old. This is the age when the baby has finished the primary vaccine series and the baby's immune system has developed enough that he won't get sick as much. Up until the age of two years, as many as 6-7 upper respiratory infections per season, are considered normal. This number slows down after the baby turns two years. This is a good age to continue, in earnest, potty training for the baby. A good rule of thumb is to see when the baby starts telling you after he wets himself. Then you know that the baby is becoming conscious of the peeing and pooping sensations. Or the baby goes and hides behind a sofa to poop. The best way I tell parents to start training is to put a cotton underwear on the baby (not a pull up as the baby cannot differentiate between a diaper and a pull up). Put on the underwear in the morning, after the baby has eaten breakfast, for a period of one hour. During that hour, put the baby on the potty every fifteen minutes to see if she will pee on it (peeing on the potty comes first, then pooping). If she pees on the potty you clap and praise her. If she pees in the underwear you just clean her and change her underwear without any fuss. If the baby stays dry during that one hour and pees only on the potty consistently for a week then you start increasing that hour to two and so on. The good thing about this approach is that if the baby starts to resist then you can back off and try again in a few weeks. It is important to not force the baby into doing something when she is not ready for it. Some babies resist pooping on the toilet which leads to constipation. If that happens, back off from training for a few days and put the baby on a stool softener like Pedi lax for a few days. As part of the 2-year-old checkup, baby's hemoglobin is checked in the office via a finger prick. It is important to maintain a hemoglobin of at least twelve for our children, because low hemoglobin (anemia) can lead to slower mental development. Even good eaters don't get enough Iron in their diets. That is why it is important to supplement with multi-vitamins with Iron. By this age baby has about sixteen teeth and needs teeth brushed twice a day with non-fluoride toothpaste. Fluoride supplements or treatments can be given at the pediatrician's office. Once the baby turns two years old the well check visits get spaced out to once a year.

14

Fun times ahead!
3-4 years pre-school years.

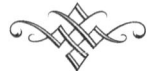

Congratulations parents; you have survived the terrible twos! The preschool years are as much fun as the toddler years were. Your baby finally starts listening to you! The baby's vocabulary takes off to about 300-500 words and the baby can talk in complete sentences. By the time the baby turns four years old the baby's speech is understandable 100% to strangers. The baby also has a fantasy friend at this point who regularly visits your child and talks and plays with her. The baby can throw and kick a ball and ride a tricycle. The child can kick a ball forward, hop on one foot, catch a thrown ball, draw circles and squares and draw a person with 2-4 body parts. The 3-4-year-old learns by exploring. They can focus well on simple tasks at hand and think creatively. It is important for parents to not force-feed the baby no matter how picky they think the child is being. She should be allowed to feed herself in a high chair with parents around to watch her. Just make sure to offer baby a variety of foods. Studies have shown that the more variety is offered to babies, the better eaters they eventually become. When babies are fed by parents, they invariably lose the ability to stop eating when they are full, causing them to over eat, which fosters obesity in later life. Early childhood studies have shown that most four-year-olds are ready to start preschool. Most states now pay for the four-year-old's schooling which is called Voluntary Pre-Kindergarten (VPK). This is a good way to get children ready for Kindergarten. I encourage all my parents to enroll their kids in the VPK program if offered in their area. Also when the four-year-old comes in to see me for his annual physical we administer the booster vaccines also. That way the child will get the boosters before starting the VPK.

15

Official start of school!

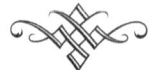

The five-year-old milestone is important in more than one way. It heralds the official start of school years for the child but also indicates the first step into independence away from the primary caregiver (mostly moms) for most children. The most important indicators of success in KG for children are good social, listening and language skills. Girls typically are a little bit ahead of boys in all the above parameters. Boys catch up fairly quickly. This is the age when eating habits also improve and toddler, frequent snack-based eating is replaced by big kid, three meals a day eating pattern. Most picky eaters, when left to their own devices, start eating better as they see other kids eat independently around them during snack time and lunch time. This is their first exposure to peer pressure! The five-year-olds also start more hands-on, book-based learning. I always tell my parents to get the children ready for kindergarten by taking them to visit the school beforehand, or enroll in the summer reading programs offered at the school. Also parents and older siblings should start talking about the school in a positive fashion beforehand! All children require their booster vaccines and physicals before registering for school. All children get evaluated, upon entry into kindergarten, for speech fluency. Any delays as perceived by the teacher or the evaluator get referred for speech evaluation and therapy. I always screen for any speech problems at every well visit with me so that any delays can be referred as soon as possible.

16

6-7-year-old child!

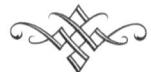

Once first grade starts, the child's learning takes off exponentially. The attention span and learning speed increases differently for each child and any deviation should not be perceived as abnormal right away. Any persistent problems in learning over time, of course, need to be discussed with first the teacher and then the pediatrician. The first and second grader is reading fluently. By second grade most kids are doing simple addition and subtraction and reading to learn (before this they were learning to read). The social skills have improved tremendously and the concept of "best friends" evolves. This is also a good age to start introducing a second language to the child at school. A lot of kids are exposed to a second language at home anyway. But formal introduction of a second language at school is also recommended. The eating habits are still evolving. It is very important for parents and caregivers who are responsible for feeding children, like grandparents, to be guided to ensure that they offer children healthy snacks like nuts, fresh fruits and vegetables 2-3 times a day. Sodas, juices and juice drinks are strictly discouraged (even 100% juice) as they foster obesity in children. The best hydration fluid is water for all of us. Most school lunch menus are subpar and offer unhealthy choices like hamburgers and pizzas. I usually encourage my families to pack lunch from home with whole grain bread, cheese and meat like turkey or chicken breast, water bottles and a piece of fruit. Children between the ages of 4-10 years require 1000 mg of calcium plus Vitamin D to maintain healthy bones and teeth. For children, milk, yogurt and cheese are the main sources of calcium and vitamin D intake. Each child should consume about twelve ounces of 1% milk, one box of low fat yogurt and one slice of low fat cheese per day to adequately supply the recommended amount. Remember to offer small portion sizes at each meal. Also the children should be given one chewable multi-vitamin with Iron per day plus a fish oil tablet per day. The children should be physically active every day for at least two hours. This includes riding bikes, skipping rope, soccer, football etc. In today's busy parental schedule often the kids' outside active time gets eliminated. I always emphasize the importance of this to my families. Screen time (TV and video games) should be discouraged during week days and no more than two hours per day on weekends. I also discourage my parents from placing TV or computers in the kids' bedrooms.

17

8-15-year-old visit!

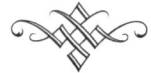

This is the age for rapid physical and intellectual growth for the kids. I like to see my kids for regular physical check-ups every year. Most kids will grow about two inches in height and gain 5-7 pounds in weight per year. Girls will start what is called pre-pubertal growth phase around age ten years (may start as early as seven years). The girls will gain a little weight and become very self-conscious as they start developing some breast tissue around age 9-10 years. The average age for girls to start their periods is about one year after this. The girls undergo what is called the peak height velocity (which means they grow the fastest) about six months before their periods start. For most girls their growth slows down after their periods start. On average, girls continue to grow about half an inch to an inch per year for about 3-4 years after the onset of periods. It is important for the family to be supportive of the girls during this period of rapid physical growth and change. It is also important for families to realize that for the first 2-3 years after the onset of menstruation, girls can have irregular periods. I always reassure my families that it is a normal part of hormonal maturation and given time (usually two years) the periods will become more regular. This irregularity does not need to be treated. Girls who are physically active can have irregular periods for a longer period. Boys usually start their puberty around age twelve when their testicles increase in size, other signs follow and boys will have their peak height velocity at an average age of 13-14 years. Boys will continue to grow for about five years after they hit the peak height velocity versus girls who will grow for about 3-4 years. Sometimes boys will develop a temporary enlargement of their breast tissue which subsides after a few months. This is also normal. If concerned consult your pediatrician. Another universal phenomenon is the development of acne on the face and upper back (sometimes neck) of adolescents. Teaching proper skin care to both boys and girls is very important. They need to clean their skin with a good cleanser and hydrate with a good moisturizer every day.

19

16-20-year-olds!

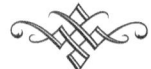

This is the time for more intellectual and emotional growth as physical growth is either totally or mostly complete. The level of cognitive development at the start of this age range gives us a good indication of how mature our youngster will eventually become. Girls will attain emotional maturity earlier than boys easily by about three years. Most kids are starting to drive at this age and perceive themselves as immortal, so it is important to provide them with the proper safety information and driver instructions. Kids are also dating at this age and, unfortunately, no matter how much we, as parents dislike it, some of them become sexually active. I always discuss this with my patients and emphasize their proper usage of barrier contraceptives, like condoms, (usually without the parents being in the room). Parents need to discuss safety and health with their kids in a nonjudgmental fashion and encourage open discussion. Kids also experiment a lot in this age and will sometimes succumb to peer pressure for hasty and ill-advised entry into drugs. I advise my parents to stay supportive and indulge in open dialogues with their kids about the evils of drugs and early sex and most kids will eventually take the right route with family support. Team sports are a very healthy form of entertainment and building self-esteem and self-discipline in this age and I strongly recommend it for both sexes. Plus kids should be encouraged to partake of chores around the house and also be working part time somewhere and volunteer in the community. These extracurricular activities enhance the kid's self-esteem and keep them busy. Volunteering also teaches young people empathy for their fellow human beings and makes them realize that they are part of the larger community outside their home. I also discuss gender/sexual orientation issues and making good choices for choosing life partners.

20

21-26 years.

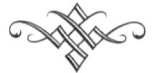

As mentioned in the beginning of this book, I will usually continue to see my patients till the age of 26 years, unless the kids get married or move away or they prefer to not be seen by a pediatrician. This is the age of young adulthood when kids will usually come to see me without their parents. Aside from any physical ailment, I continue to see them every year for a thorough physical exam. I again discuss safety and making healthy choices in their daily lives like eating healthy, staying away from drugs and alcohol and abstinence. I teach my girl patients breast self-exam and boys how to perform a testicular exam, both important tools for early cancer screenings. Most kids have moved out of the parent's houses for work and school at this age so I like to discuss with them how to choose an appropriate roommate for optimum functioning.

Conclusion

So here I am at the end of my very brief treatise into the wonderful, sometimes stressful, yet ever rewarding world of parenthood. I have tried to keep it brief and meaningful so that parents of kids of all ages can draw upon it as a source of quick reference. This book by no means replaces your child's wonderful pediatrician who is your full time partner in raising your child. Remember, there is always more than one correct way of doing things and we are all human beings first and foremost and can make mistakes. There is no such thing as a perfect parent. Trust your instincts, do your best, maintain a sense of humor and pray and you will do fine. God bless!

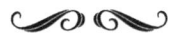

Appendix

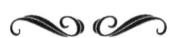

Hepatitis B
- BIRTH
- 2 MOS.
- 6 MOS.

DTAP (Diphtheria, Tetanus And Pertussis)
- 2 MOS.
- 4 MOS.
- 6 MOS.
- 15-18 MOS

TDAP (Booster)
- 11 YRS

Hemophilus Influenzae Type B
- 2 MOS.
- 4 MOS.
- 6 MOS.
- 15-18 MOS.

POLIO
- 2 MOS.
- 4 MOS.
- 6 MOS.

Pneumococcal Vaccine
- 2 MOS.
- 4 MOS.
- 6 MOS.
- 15-18 MOS.

ROTAVIRUS
- 2 MOS.
- 4 MOS.
- 6 MOS.

Measles, Mumps and Rubella
- 12 MOS.
- 4-6 YRS

VARICELLA
- 12 MOS.
- 4-6 YRS

MENACTRA
- 11 YRS
- 16 YRS

Human Papilloma Virus
- STARTS @ 9 YRS (GIRLS)
- STARTS @ 11 YRS (BOYS)

3 Vaccine series.